Orestes M. Brands

Good Health for Children

In easy lessons upon food, drink, air, and exercise

Orestes M. Brands

Good Health for Children
In easy lessons upon food, drink, air, and exercise

ISBN/EAN: 9783337393496

Printed in Europe, USA, Canada, Australia, Japan

Cover: Foto ©Lupo / pixelio.de

More available books at **www.hansebooks.com**

GOOD HEALTH FOR CHILDREN,

IN

EASY LESSONS UPON FOOD, DRINK, AIR, AND EXERCISE.

BY

ORESTES M. BRANDS,

SUPERINTENDENT OF SCHOOLS, PATERSON, N.J.; AUTHOR OF "LESSONS ON
THE HUMAN BODY" AND "HEALTH LESSONS FOR BEGINNERS."

REVISED EDITION

LEACH, SHEWELL, AND SANBORN,

BOSTON AND NEW YORK.

PREFACE.

In the preparation of this little book my object has been to select the most essential points in the personal care of the health, and to speak *in a known tongue* about them to young children.

Technical terms have been regarded as husks and studiously avoided. Simple, familiar language has been chosen as the medium of communication with the mind of the child.

How to teach the younger children the essentials of physiology and hygiene is a question which has recently received much consideration. The easy, conversational style of the text in the following pages is intended to be suggestive to the teacher. The facts, the phenomena, are what the children should understand, and these can be communicated in the simplest language.

Especial prominence has been given to the baneful effects of alcohol and tobacco, and this portion of the subject is also treated simply and cogently.

It is recommended that the pupils should frequently be required to write short compositions
upon selected topics; and that the script inter-
spersed in the lessons be written upon the black-
board, and copied upon slates. The teacher can
invest every topic with greater interest by making
it a subject of conversation and explanation.

This little volume, having been revised in accord-
ance with valuable suggestions of Mrs. Mary H.
Hunt, Superintendent of the Department of Scientific
Instruction of the National W. C. T. U., receives the
approval of that earnest and influential organization
whose mission it is not alone to reform the adult,
but to so educate the child that he may escape the
snares and allurements of "King Alcohol."

O. M. B.

CONTENTS.

6 CONTENTS.

GOOD HEALTH FOR CHILDREN.

LESSON I.

LEARNING TO KEEP A HEALTHY BODY.

1. A few years ago you were a helpless babe. Of course you could breathe, and cry, and swallow milk; but you did not know what it was all about, after all. The little kittens could perform the same acts and others as well; and so, while they knew as much as you did, they were not so helpless.

2. Your good mother, father, or grandmother had to take constant care of you. If they had not known how to feed, bathe, and clothe you properly, you would not now be alive and well. The better you were cared for, the stronger you became.

3. As you grew a little older and began to move about, there was danger of your doing some great harm to yourself. The fire might burn you, the knife might cut you, the fork might pierce your eyes, the pepper might fly into them or get into your mouth, or you might tumble down stairs! You were very apt to put into your mouth unfit food or poisonous stuff that, by accident, was left where you could

7

get it. You were yet too young to know the danger
in all these things.

4. Little by little you learned to avoid some
things which would injure you; but you did not
always know why. You believed what your parents
told you. What do you think would have happened
to you if you had not? You might have been very
badly injured, or even killed? Yes, indeed you
would have been.

5. You are now old enough to take more care of
yourselves. You are not now always in the house
with mother. Often, when you are away from her,
you need to know what to avoid; if you do not
know, the harm will be done.

6. Perhaps you know some one who spoiled or
broke his pretty toy or handsome watch, just because
he did not know what would injure it. Well, the
toy or the watch could be repaired, if not too badly
broken, or a new one could be bought. How will it
be if children do not learn how to take care of their
bodies and their health? Can they have them repaired when they are much injured? No, not always.
Often they will have to live with broken-down bodies
all the rest of their lives. But likely they will not
live to be men or women. They cannot get new
bodies, and begin again, in the right way.

7. You should learn that some careless, bad habits
will show the harm they do at once, and that some
do their evil work slowly. It is certain that the
injury will be felt when you are older, if not just

now. What is the best thing to do? Why, to learn now to avoid danger. Now copy this motto neatly on your slates, and try to keep it in mind: —

I should study how to keep the health the kind Creator has given me.

LESSON II.

OUR BODIES.

1. What is this body, this "I"? Well, let us think a little. You know that it breathes, eats, thinks, talks, moves about, and that it has learned how to do many things. Part of the time, as you know, it is tired, and then it rests and sleeps. Even when asleep it breathes, and so it needs pure air all the time. It is a very wonderful, living machine!

2. The softer parts of this machine — your body — are built upon or within a frame of bones, called the skeleton. The frame and all upon it and within it grow larger and stronger when good care is taken of them.

3. There are a great many bones in the frame-work, — not less than two hundred and eight in number. They are joined together very curiously. All are kept in their places by bands and cords that hold them quite firmly. Nothing ever made by man can compare with it in workmanship.

4. Some of the bones are joined so as to move like the hinges of a door. Some, which have ball-shaped ends, fit into sockets in other bones, and can be swung about in any direction. You notice how smoothly the joints move. One bone does not grate upon another. No, because the ends of the bones are covered with firm, smooth gristle; and besides, a kind of oil comes out into the joints and keeps them in good order.

5. Away at the top of the frame are the bones of the head or skull. These are rounded and joined together so as to form a hollow place for the brain, which is soft and needs to be lodged in a safe place.

6. The head rests upon a set of bones called the spine, or backbone. Here are twenty-four bones placed one upon another, and so bound together that it is hard to separate them. Yet this column of bones can be bent in all directions. Between the bones are little pads or cushions of gristle. These pads are springy; and when you walk, run, or jump. they save the brain from rough jars.

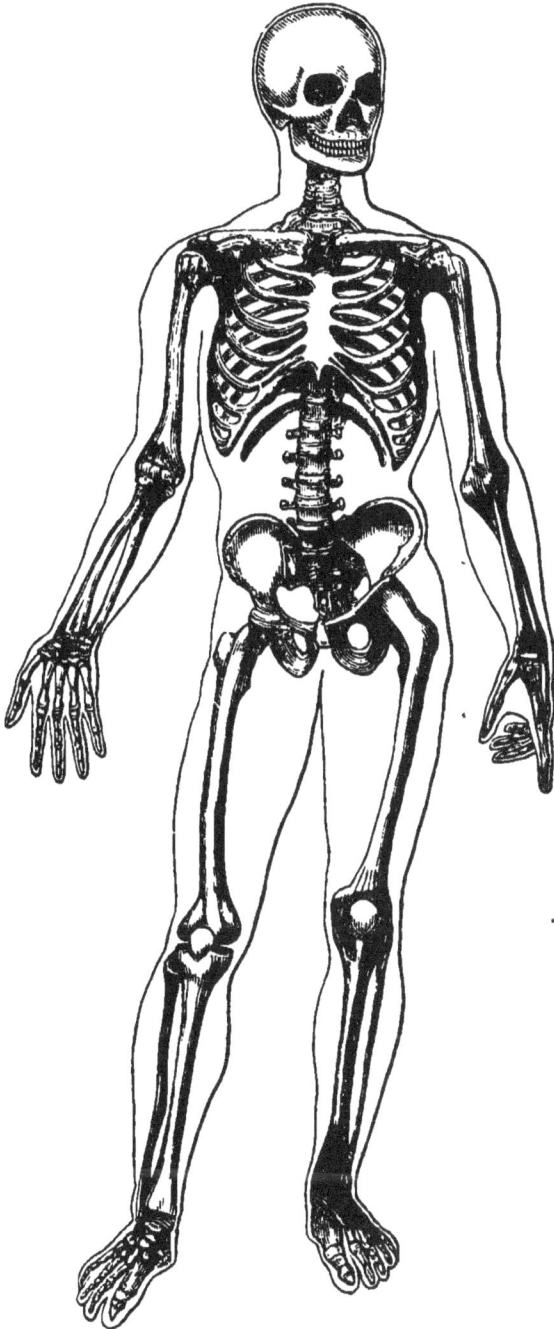

SKELETON. — The Outer Lines show the Form of the Human Body when the Skeleton is clothed with Flesh.

7. The large, barrel-shaped part of your body is called the *trunk*. It is not solid like the trunk of a tree. Indeed, there are two rooms in it. Let us notice these rooms, and see what they have in them.

8. The curved ribs go round the upper part of the trunk like hoops around a barrel. They are joined to the backbone behind, and to the breastbone in front. Here, then, we have a cage or room, and in it are the heart and lungs. This upper room has a fleshy floor, and below it is the lower room of the trunk. In the lower room are the stomach, liver, and bowels. The upper room is called the *chest*, and the lower one the *abdomen*. Has the trunk limbs? Yes; your arms and legs are its limbs.

9. The framework of your body is hidden from sight. It is covered by muscles which are fastened to the bones. Muscles are the lean flesh, and they are wrapped about the bones in very curious ways. Last of all, the soft skin is spread over the muscles and covers the whole body.

10. You can think, then, of your body as having in it many kinds of machinery, all working together. In it is machinery for eating, drinking, breathing, and moving the blood. Yes, and machinery to move the whole body or any part of it.

11. When all the other machinery is in good order, the thinking machinery always works well. Here are a few short directions for keeping all the machinery in good order. Copy them very neatly. You will soon learn more about them.

Keep the whole skin very clean.

Breathe pure air; eat wholesome food.

Take regular exercise in the fresh air.

LESSON III.

MORE ABOUT THE FRAMEWORK.

1. We can take much better care of anything, and keep it much longer for use, when we know of what it is made. We need to know what things will bear. The other day a large boy climbed into a baby carriage. He now knows that the little carriage would not bear so much weight, for its springs are broken, and its frame is bent out of shape. Well, as your bodies have frames and springs, it will be

wise to learn of what they are made, and what they
will bear. The frame is made of bone? Yes, but
what is bone made of?

2. Let us go to the butcher and get a bone, just
taken from the meat. It is not an old, dry bone.
It looks pink, and is firm and tough. Now put the
bone into the fire, and let it burn awhile. Well,
the bone has been burned. What now? Why,
the bone is just as large as it was, but it is very
white, and not nearly so heavy. Is it tough? No,
for see how brittle! There is nothing left of it but
lime.

3. You got two bones just alike? Well, we will
soak this one for a few days in some acid. We
must be patient. Now let us see what has happened
to it. Does it look like the burned bone? No, the
lime is dissolved out of it. It is just as large, and
of the same shape. But see! it is like tough jelly
or gristle. It bends very easily, and if it were long
enough, we could tie it in a knot. We have found
that bones are made of lime, and of tough animal
matter, or jelly.

4. Now, we know that the lime in the bones
makes them hard and firm, and the jelly-like part
makes them tough and slightly elastic. So, if your
bones had no lime in them they would bend like
gristle. They would neither support your weight,
nor keep your body in shape. If they were made
entirely of lime they would be too brittle, and would
soon be broken into many small pieces.

I must not let my bones bend out of shape; for they may stay so.

5. The bones of children are not so hard and firm as those of old people. As the bones grow older they become harder and more brittle, because there is more lime and less jelly in them. The bones of children will often bend a little without breaking. You know that a green twig will bend without breaking, but that a dry one will snap off. Well, your bones are like the green twig. But you know that if you keep the green twig bent while it is growing larger and thicker, it will then remain bent. Will your bones do so? Yes, certainly, if you are not very careful.

6. Children who do not stand and sit erect, who do not keep their heads up, and their shoulders thrown back, often have bent bones. Sometimes the bones bend in upon the machinery in the trunk and do much harm. How sad it is to see boys and girls getting misshapen frames from bad habits!

Would you like to write a letter to your teacher about what you have read in this lesson?

LESSON IV.

TAKING CARE OF THE BONY FRAME.

1. If the frame of a house is not strong, and so gets out of shape, or if any of its timbers bend or twist, other parts will be injured. The walls will crack, and the doors will be pressed upon so that they cannot swing. If the frame of a machine becomes bent, its wheels and cogs cannot move as they should.

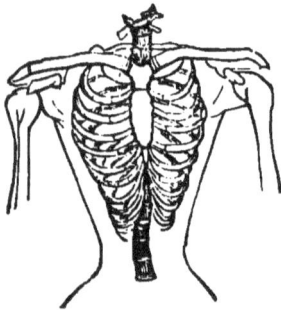

2. So easily do the bones of children yield to pressure, that they are often bent out of shape by careless habits. Bad positions in sitting and standing, and tight clothing, are the things you should avoid. No part of the frame can be bent out of shape or crowded out of place without doing more or less injury to the body. Sometimes poor health and early death are caused in this way.

3. If the bones are crowded out of place, they must go somewhere. If the ribs are pressed upon by tight clothing, they will go inward and crowd the lungs by making the chest too small. Look at this picture and see how the ribs may be pressed inward in this way. The heart, stomach, and liver will also be crowded, and so cannot do their work well.

Breathing, blood-making, and blood-moving are thus hindered by tight clothing at the chest and waist.

4. Children often sit at their desks in school, or stand in their classes in a stooping position. It soon becomes a habit to stoop over, or to bend sidewise. The bones of the back, and the pads between them, grow and harden in this position. Yes, and some of the muscles are strained and weakened so that they cannot hold the backbone upright. You should sit and stand erect, and should not let your shoulders droop forward. An ill-shaped backbone and hollow chest make a weak body.

5. Your desk should not be so high as to cause you to raise one shoulder higher than the other when you write, nor so low that you stoop over it. Your chair should not be so high that you cannot rest your feet upon the floor, else you cannot keep erect. If the seat is too low, the back and shoulders will be strained.

6. Some joints are quite easily injured, and the bones pushed or twisted out of place. Children who are rough in playing may tear or strain a cord at a joint. Such an injury is called a *sprain*, and is sometimes more painful than a broken bone.

7. Our feet should be as free to move and to grow as our hands. How silly it is to crowd and twist their bones out of shape by wearing short, narrow, high-heeled boots and shoes! Just think! Five toes crowded into a space not wide enough for three! Yes, and the weight of the body thrown upon the

poor, cramped toes by the high heels! Corns and
bunions also begin to make trouble for the pinched
feet, and the nails cut into the flesh. Don't like to
walk? No wonder! Feel cross, also? Why, of
course!

8. You know that drunken people often fall and
break their bones, and you may think that this is the
only way in which the liquors that make people
drunk can injure the framework. Let us think
about it. The bones are alive as well as the muscles
and other soft parts of the body. The blood flows
through them, feeds them, and builds them up.

It cannot do this if it does not contain the kind
of food needed by the bones. When a person drinks
wine, beer, cider or stronger liquors the poison which
these drinks contain gets into his blood and makes
it bad. Such blood does not carry to the bones the
food they need to make them grow or keep them
strong and well. The name of the poison is alcohol.
In another chapter you will learn more about it and
what it does to those who drink it. The use of
tobacco also makes bad blood. Doctors say that it
stunts the growth and that no boy should use it if
he wishes to have a fine, manly form.

Alcohol is a poison.
Use neither alcohol nor tobacco.

.

LESSON V.

A SHORT STORY ABOUT ALCOHOL AND TOBACCO.

1. Some of the first white men who came to this country brought strong, fiery liquors with them on their ships. They gave some of this liquor to the Indians they met at a certain place. The Indians drank part of the liquor, and soon became very merry. They danced and sang, and felt very gay. Nothing like this had ever happened to them before.

2. They drank more of the hot-tasting drink, and soon began to stagger and fall. At last they could stand no longer, and all fell asleep upon the ground. When they awakened, after a long sleep, their eyes were red, their heads ached, and all felt very miserable. How very thirsty they all were! It seemed to them that the white men's strong drink had burned their throats and stomachs. They all agreed that they had drunk " Fire-water."

3. Alcohol does look like water, and it has a hot, biting taste. Indeed, when it is taken clear, it burns the mouth, throat, and stomach like fire. No wonder that the Indians called it *fire-water!* It may be that they had drunk either *brandy* or *whiskey*, *gin* or *rum*, any of which is about half alcohol.

4. It is the alcohol in these that makes people drunk and takes away their senses. Alcohol is a fiery poison, and when people once begin to take it, they often become unable to stop taking it. It makes slaves of them, and often leads them to do horrible deeds. In other lessons you will learn how it harms the body of any one who is so foolish as to drink it.

ALCOHOL A POISON.

5. A cat or dog may be killed by causing it to drink a small quantity of alcohol. A boy once drank whiskey from a flask he had found, and died within a few hours. His death was caused by the alcohol in the whiskey. Many people have been poisoned by liquors containing alcohol.

6. But why has not every one who has drunk beer or whiskey been killed by them if they are poisons. The answer to that question is easy. A little of some kinds of poisons will not kill at once. Some people drink wine and beer every day and are not killed by them just then because they get only a little of the alcohol at a time. But that does not prove that alcohol is harmless; it is a poison, and will injure the health and shorten the lives of those who take it in this way. It is thought that alcoholic drinks, as a rule, take from six to twenty-six years from the lives of those who use them.[1]

---

[1] Life-insurance companies make a close study of the death rate among all classes of people so that they may know who are likely to be short-lived. In this way they are able to predict very nearly the number of deaths that will occur among any class of people within a given time. Neison's statistics show that a temperate person at the

7. Now let us hear the rest of the story. At another place the white men saw the Indians do something which astounded them. What was it? Well, the Indians puffed smoke from their mouths and noses, as though on fire within! They were smoking the dried leaves of the *tobacco* plant.

8. The new-comers did not know anything about tobacco, but the Indians soon taught them how to use it. No doubt these men were made deathly sick by the tobacco, because it has that effect upon people the first time they use it.

Alcohol and Tobacco cause disease and shorten life.

9. In tobacco there is a very powerful poison called *nicotine*. A few drops of it will kill a dog, and just as few would kill a child. When tobacco is smoked or chewed, nicotine gets into the blood through the thin lining skin of the mouth. Some of it is swallowed into the stomach. It spoils the blood,

---

age of twenty years has the life-expectancy of 44 years ; at thirty years of age, 36 years ; at forty, 28 years; at fifty, 22 years; at sixty, 14 years. The intemperate person at twenty has an expectancy of 15 years — one-third that of the abstainer; at thirty, 13 years; at forty, 11 years ; at fifty, 10 years; and at sixty, 9 years. The average duration of life after commencing the use of alcoholic drinks is, among mechanics and laborers, 18 years ; store-keepers and men of leisure, 15 years; and among females, 14 years.

makes the stomach weak, and causes loss of appetite for food. Sometimes it causes cancer in the mouth or throat.

10. Tobacco is a great enemy of young, growing bodies. Boys, look out! It injures the heart, and weakens the nerves and muscles. It is very harmful to boys. Many are stunting their bodies and their minds by using tobacco. Don't be deceived by it. It may not seem to hurt some who use it, but after a while its bad work will be seen.

11. Alcohol and tobacco are much alike in some of their bad effects. Both have a strange power to make people want more of them, and this appetite often grows so strong that the mind cannot master it. The only safe way is *never to venture to use either of them.*

The bones require exercise to make them healthy.

The blood runs through the bones.

Alcohol and tobacco poison the blood and injure the bones.

12. The poor, wretched, drunken men and women you may have seen were once bright, healthy children like you. No one could have made them believe that they would become drunkards, and lose their health, property, and good names. They never meant to fall so low. They thought that they could venture to drink without taking too much. You see what a sad mistake they made! It is never safe to begin the use of either alcoholic drinks or tobacco, for it is their nature to make those who take them want more.

TEST QUESTIONS FOR REVIEW.

THE BONY FRAME.

Lesson I. — Who took care of you when you were a babe? What are you now old enough to learn? What may happen if you do not learn how to care for your health? What is said about some bad habits?

Lesson II. — What does your body need constantly? What is the skeleton? How may you make your body grow larger and stronger? What binds the bones together? Tell about the kinds of joints, and how they move. Where is your brain, and what is it for? Tell what you have read about the backbone. Tell about the trunk and its rooms. What covers the framework? What kinds of machinery are in your body? When does the thinking machinery work best?

Lesson III. — Why should we know of what things are made? Of what two things are bones made? Tell about burning a bone and soaking one in acid. Of what use is lime to the bone? The jelly? How are the bones of children? How may they get bent out of shape? What harm would this do? What kind of blood must a person have in order that his bones may grow? What drinks make the blood bad? Why should not boys use tobacco?

Lesson IV. — What bad habits may put your bones out of shape? What harm will this do? What if the ribs are pressed upon by tight clothing? What can you tell about stooping in sitting? How should you sit and stand? How high should your desk be? Your chair? Why? How may joints be injured in play? Tell about tight boots and shoes and the harm they do. How do alcohol and tobacco injure the bones? What harm does tobacco do to the frames of boys who use it?

Lesson V. — Tell the story of the Iudians and the strong drink. What is alcohol like? What would it do if it was drunk clear? What is it that makes people drunk? What harm does alcohol do to those who drink it? What shows that alcohol is a poison? What may alcohol do to the lives of people? Tell the story about the Indians and their tobacco. What poison is in tobacco? How does the poison of tobacco get into the blood? What hurt does it do? In what way does tobacco injure young people? What strange power have alcohol and tobacco? What is the best way to be safe from them?

—◦◦◦—

LESSON VI.

HOW ALCOHOL IS OBTAINED FROM FRUITS.

1. Here is a ripe, rosy apple. How full of juice it is! It tastes as if it had been sweetened with sugar. There is sugar in its juice; but no one put it there. As the apple grew and ripened the sugar formed in its juice.

2. When apples are ripe and sound they are good. We like to eat them. They are sometimes dried. Apple that has been quickly dried in the right way looks white as it does when first cut. The water in its juice has been dried out. In this way apple may be made to keep for a long time. When such dried apple is soaked in water it may be cooked for food as fresh apples are.

3. Every year quantities of apples which might be used in useful ways are worse than destroyed by being made into a dangerous liquid for people to drink. This liquid is called cider. You remember there was a poison called alcohol in the white man's drink that led the Indians to name it "Fire-water." This same poison is in the cider very soon after it is made. How does it get there? Does anybody put it in? No, it gets there in a curious way. Men first grind the apples and then squeeze out their juice. There is water and sugar in this juice when it first leaves the apples; but when it has stood for a few hours in a warm place the sugar begins to change to alcohol. What makes it change? Something called a ferment.

4. You have bright, young eyes. When you look out into the air you think you see everything that is there. But if you were to look at the air through the microscope you would see many things that your naked eyes cannot. Your teacher will tell you what a microscope is. What things would you thus see? One of them might be a ferment.

5. A ferment is so very, very small you cannot see it with the naked eye. Ferments often rest on the skin or stems of fruit. From these or from the air these ferments are easily carried into the apple juice when it is squeezed out. There the ferments change the sugar of the apple juice to alcohol.

6. Although you cannot see these ferments with
the naked eye, you may know when they are present
in the apple juice by the little bubbles which rise to
the top of the barrel or vessel containing the cider.
What causes these bubbles?

7. The ferments in the apple juice are not only
turning its sugar to alcohol, but to a gas [1] also, that
rises in bubbles. These bubbles break at the top and
let the gas go off into the air. They carry a froth to
the top of the cider. Whenever you see the bubbles
of gas rising in cider you may know that the ferments
are at work in it, changing the sugar into a gas and
alcohol. This gas does no harm because nearly all
of it passes out of the apple juice.

8. Does the alcohol pass out of the cider with
the gas? No, the alcohol stays in the cider, and as
alcohol is a poison, it turns the cider to a poisonous
drink. From the moment the ferments begin to
work in the cider it begins to be an unsafe drink.
In a few hours after apple juice is pressed out alcohol
is usually found in it. Each day it contains a little
more alcohol than it did the day before. Whoever
drinks of it from time to time as it is growing stronger
with alcohol, is getting more and more of this dangerous poison.

9. It is the nature of alcohol to make any one who
drinks it want more and still more alcohol, and to
care more for drinking liquors that contain alcohol

[1] Carbonic acid gas.

than for anything else. A person who likes alcohol as well as this, and thus keeps drinking it, is called a drunkard.

10. Many a man who is a drunkard got the liking for the drinks that have ruined him by drinking cider. The alcohol in the cider made him want more alcohol. After a while he craved other drinks which were still stronger of alcohol than cider is. The more of these he drank the more he wanted, and the worse his condition became.

11. Because there is alcohol in cider, we cannot be sure that any one who drinks it will not become a drunkard. It is the nature of alcohol to make drunkards. Besides injuring the health, cider, and other liquors also, often make their drinkers cross, selfish, unkind, and careless about doing right, before they get to be drunkards.

LESSON VII.

WINE: ALCOHOL FROM GRAPES, ETC.

1. Grapes as they hang in large ripe clusters on the vines or from dishes of fruit upon the table are very beautiful. They are as good to eat as they are beautiful to look at. But every year tons of grapes, like the apples, are worse than wasted to make another dangerous drink called wine.

2. To make wine, the juice of grapes is crushed out and left standing in warm air. You remember that the ferments changed the apple juice, and that they often rest on the skins and stems of fruit. From there or from the air they quickly get into this grape juice. In a short time they make a great change in the nature of this juice, which was so sweet and good while in the grape. Bubbles of a gas[1] rise to the top, showing that the sugar of the juice is being destroyed, and alcohol is taking its place. The alcohol does not go out of the grape juice with the gas, but stays in it, turning the juice of the beautiful grapes to a poison.

3. There are people who think that cider and wine must be good because the apples and grapes from which they are made are good. You have learned that this is not true because the ferments change the sugar of the fruit juices to a poison which remains in the liquid, making the whole poisonous.

4. In countries where much wine is made many people become drunkards by using it. During the wine-making season in some places many of the people are in a drunken state much of the time.[2] The alcohol in the wine affects them so, that the more they take the more they want. It is its nature to do this.

---

[1] Carbonic acid gas.

[2] The Rev. J. G. Cochran, who for a long time was a resident missionary in Persia, speaking of wine-drinking in that country, says, " In the wine-making season the whole village of male adults will be habitually intoxicated for a month or six weeks."

For this reason those who drink wine may soon come to like liquors that contain more alcohol than there is in wine. You should never drink wine. No one can drink it without being in danger of becoming a drunkard.

5. Wine is sometimes made from other kinds of fruits and berries, such as currants, raspberries, and elderberries. All such wines are unsafe drinks, for the ferments work on the sugar in the liquid juice of such fruits and change it into the poison alcohol.

6. There are many kinds of ferments besides those that turn the sugar in fruit juices to alcohol. One kind enters into cider and wine when they are allowed to stand open to the air and changes the alcohol which they contain into a sharp acid. This makes vinegar. There is no alcohol in vinegar.

7. You see from this that ferments may do both good and harm. They are very strange things and we do not begin to know all that we hope to learn about them. But this much we know, — they make great changes in the nature of the things on which they act. They change the sugar in good fruit juices to alcohol, which is a poison, and they change alcohol to vinegar, which may be used with safety as a flavoring for foods.

8. Strange as all this may seem, it is not more strange than the change which alcohol makes in the nature of most people who use it. It makes a strong man weak, a wise man foolish, a kind man cruel, and

a good man bad. But it does not make a bad man good. It makes him so much worse that he sometimes does terrible deeds that he would not think of doing if he did not use alcoholic drinks.

———

LESSON VIII.

BEER: ALCOHOL FROM GRAINS.

1. Beer is an alcoholic drink made in large quantities from grain, generally from barley. You have already seen that the little ferments will turn sugar to alcohol when they find it dissolved in water, as it is in the fruit juices; but there is no water in grain, and the hard, dry part of grain is not sugar, but is mostly starch. How can alcohol be made from such a dry grain as barley? It cannot, if it is left whole and dry; but men moisten the barley and keep it in a warm place until it sprouts or begins to grow.

2. If you ever tasted a kernel of sprouted barley you found it sweet. The sprouting turned the starch to sugar. Men grind this sprouted barley and dissolve out its sugar with water. Into this they put yeast, which is one kind of ferment, and hops for a flavor. The ferments in the yeast quickly change the sugar in this barley juice to alcohol, and to the gas that goes off into the air, while the alcohol stays in the beer. People who think beer a healthful drink, because it is made from grain, are greatly mistaken; it is poisoned by alcohol. A wise man has truly said, " As much flour as can lie on the point of a table knife has more nourishment in it than eight quarts of the best beer." [1]

3. Flour made from grain is of great value for food, but beer made from the same kind of grain is a poisonous drink. The ferments which produced the beer changed the whole nature of the barley juice. They turned the food that would have nourished the body into a poison that does it harm.

4. People who drink beer often grow very fat. They think from this that the beer is good for them. But such people are mistaken. They are seldom as strong or well as those who drink no liquors containing alcohol. They often grow very ill from slight causes, and sometimes die from the effect of cuts and hurts that would have soon healed if made upon persons whose blood had not been poisoned by beer. Beer drinking tends to make one's mind coarse and bad. Many a cruel deed has been done by those whose minds have been hardened by beer.

Beer made at home, by allowing a sweet liquid to ferment, also contains alcohol and should never be drunk.

5. Some drinks contain more alcohol than others. Brandy contains more than wine; whiskey, more than beer. Rum, gin, brandy and whiskey are about one-

---

[1] Liebig.

half alcohol. They are made by separating the alcohol from a portion of the water in fermented liquids.[1]

6. These strong drinks do more harm than wine or beer because they contain so much more alcohol. Drinks containing alcohol have ruined many thousands of people.

7. It is important for you to remember that it is the nature of a little alcohol to create an appetite for more. You will be less apt to care for the stronger liquors if you never drink beer, wine or cider. If you begin to use cider, beer or wine, you cannot tell how soon you may form the dreadful appetite that makes you care for nothing else so much as to get more alcohol.

TEST QUESTIONS FOR REVIEW.

Lesson VI. — What does the juice of apples contain? What drink is sometimes made from the juice of apples? When apple juice is made into cider, what becomes of the sugar it contained? What poison does cider contain very soon after it is made? What name is given to the little things that change the sugar of apple juice into alcohol? Where are ferments often found? With what can you see them? How can you know when the ferments are changing the sugar of apple juice to alcohol? Why does the gas do no harm to the cider? Why does the alcohol make it poisonous? Why should you not drink cider? What is it the nature of alcohol to do? How has many a drunkard formed his liking for alcohol? What did the alcohol in the cider make him want? How soon after it is squeezed out does cider usually contain alcohol?

Lesson VII. — What drink is made from the juice of grapes? What do the ferments do to the grape juice when it is squeezed out? Into

---

[1] This process is known as *distillation,* and the liquors thus produced are called *distilled liquors.*

what do they change the sugar of the juice? Where does the alcohol remain? What does it do to the grape juice? Why are not wine and cider as good to use as the grapes and apples from which they are made? What is true of places where wine is made? Why do those who drink wine soon come to like liquors that contain more alcohol? Of what is every one who drinks wine in danger? From what other fruits are wines sometimes made? Why are all wines unsafe drinks? What enters into cider or wine when they are allowed to remain open to the air? What change does this ferment make? Is there alcohol in vinegar? What do we know about ferments? What change does alcohol usually make in the nature of those who use it?

Lesson VIII.—What is beer? Why is beer not a healthful drink? What did a wise man once say of beer and flour? Why is flour good for food while beer, made from the same kind of grain, is a poisonous drink? What is true of people who grow fat from using beer? How does beer-drinking often affect the mind? What drinks are about one-half alcohol? Why do these drinks work more harm than beer or wine? What may be the result if you begin to use cider or wine? Why is this?

LESSON IX.

WHAT MUSCLES ARE AND WHAT THEY DO.

1. How is it that we can move about as we do? The bones are alive, but they cannot of themselves make the least movement. Raise your arm. What makes it go up? It is moved by what we call *muscles;* they pull upon the bones and raise them. Close your eyes. Muscles pulled the lids down. You breathe, and muscles move the ribs. Your heart is pumping the blood, and muscles in it give it motion. There is no motion in the body that is not made by muscles.

2. The lean meat of an ox, cow, or sheep is muscle. So when you eat beef-steak, or lean mutton, you use the muscles of these animals to make muscles for your own body. But how do the muscles pull and make parts move? Well, the muscles are made up of fine threads, laid side by side, and bound up in very thin, skin-like coverings. You can think of a piece of elastic made of fine India-rubber threads. Just so the fibres of the muscle are elastic, and when they are stretched they shrink back again. When a muscle pulls a bone, it shortens itself just as a strip of rubber does. At the ends of the muscles the threads change into slender, strong cords, which are fastened to the bones.

3. Here is a picture of the bones of an arm, and of two strong muscles. The muscle marked C shortens and pulls up the bones below the elbow

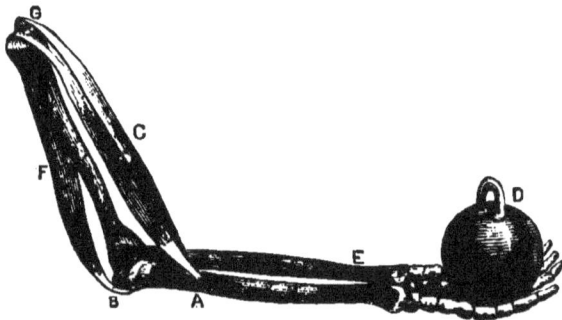

joint. The muscle marked F shortens, pulls the same bones down, and straightens the arm. Bend your arm strongly, and feel how muscle C swells out when it shortens.

4. The muscles are spread all over the frame-work, and some are inside of it as well. Some are long, and wind about the bones; others are broad and flat, and a few are shaped like rings. All of them do not move bones, but all contract to make movement. Why do so many of them end in slender cords? Well, the cords take up less room in the joints. You can see that if all the muscles that move the fingers and toes were in them, they would be very large and clumsy. So the slender cords go down from the arms and legs to the bones of the hands and feet.

5. About one-half of your body is made of muscles. Nerves and blood-vessels are everywhere in them. To have an active, healthy body, you must see to it that the muscles get plenty of exercise in play and in work.

LESSON X.

HEALTHFUL EXERCISE: HOW, WHERE, WHEN.

1. Here come the boys and girls! Their cheeks are ruddy and their eyes sparkle. How fast and deeply they breathe, and how merry they all are! What has 'caused them to look so bright, and to feel so full of life? Why, they have been exercising their muscles in the fresh air and in the sunlight, out of doors.

2. Some have been running, and others have been walking briskly about in their sports. They have been playing different games that made nearly all of their muscles move freely. Arms, legs, and trunk all came in for a share in the play, and all got it. Well, that is right; for all the muscles should have a chance to move. The strongest muscles are those that are most often used, if they are properly rested. The weakest muscles are those that are used least. Look at the stout arms of the blacksmith! See how the great muscles swell out! Yes, swinging the hammer has given them much exercise and made them so strong.

It is best to exercise in the sunlight and pure air.

3. Exercise is good for the muscles because it makes the blood flow faster through them. This makes them larger and stronger. The heart pumps faster, and away goes the blood to the lungs, and they must breathe faster and take in more air. In this way more oxygen from the air is taken into the blood in the lungs, and such blood gives more life to the whole body.

4. When is the best time for exercise? Well, not

at night. Night is the time for rest. Soon after a full meal is not a good time, for if exercise is taken then the blood will be called away from the stomach and interfere with its work. As a general rule, the morning, when the air is pure and the ground is dry, is the best time. Exercise should be taken regularly. It will not do much good unless you take it every day.

5. Tight clothing and tight shoes press upon the muscles and hinder their movements. You should let all the muscles have room to move freely. When you play and begin to feel warm, you should not throw off your coat or your sack and sit down on the ground to rest and become cool. In this way people get severe colds. Sudden cooling should be avoided after exercise.

6. In what other way can the muscles be injured? By the use of beer or wine, or other alcoholic drinks. Perhaps you have seen beer-drinkers who were very fat. They may have thought the beer did them good because it made them so fat, but their muscles were weaker instead of stronger for this fat. You remember that the muscles are lean meat. When too much fat gathers in the muscles it takes the place of some of this lean meat, and so weakens the muscle. The use of drinks that contain alcohol, especially beer, tends to an increase of useless fat in the muscles. The heart is a muscle, and alcohol can fatten and weaken it. Sometimes the tiny muscles of the blood-vessels are weakened by alcohol and burst, causing death.

7. It is thought by some that a drink of beer, wine, or whiskey, aids one in doing a piece of hard work, by making him stronger. This has been put to the test with a great deal of care, and found to be a mistake.[1] Instead of adding to the strength of the muscles such drinks make the muscles weaker.

A doctor[2] who has studied the health of soldiers says that men who use alcoholic liquors frequently, or those who use a great deal of them at a time, are the first to fail when they are put at work that requires strength or endurance. Other doctors have said the same thing.

8. Boys who smoke cigarettes are making their muscles weak. After a time smoking may not make them sick, but still it is all the time doing harm. It poisons the blood, and poor blood cannot make healthy muscles. It disturbs the heart and makes it weak. Pale faces, unhealthy skin, and puny muscles! Yes, you may soon begin to see these signs of bad health in boys who use tobacco.

9. Here is what a young man says in a letter to his friends. Boys, read it and keep it in mind: " I thought when I was a boy that being a man was to learn to drink and smoke. Unknown to my parents I formed these bad habits, and they soon took strong hold upon me. Tell the boys that smoking and drinking never made a man of any boy."

---

[1] See Richardson's " Ten Lectures on Alcohol," page 118.
[2] William H. Van Buren, M.D.

LESSON XI.

THE BRAIN AND NERVES: HOW ALCOHOL INJURES THEM.

1. All children want to grow tall, and to have strong frames and strong muscles. We have told you about some things that will make the muscles strong. Now we shall tell you more about the great enemies of the muscles. Yes, alcohol and tobacco make weak muscles. But you must learn something about nerves before you can understand this.

2. You know that you have a brain. The mind uses the brain to think with. On the next page is a picture of the brain. The bones of the skull have all been taken away. You can see the great nerve, marked SC, that goes down into the backbone. How do you suppose the mind gets to the muscles to make them work? Well, there are white thread-like cords that go from the brain, and from a large cord in the hollow of the backbone, to all parts of the body. These are *nerves*, and they act like the wires of a telegraph.

3. When the mind wishes a muscle to move, the brain sends out an order through the nerves that go to that muscle, and it does what it is bid to do. If a nerve is broken, it cannot carry orders. To do their work well, the nerves must be kept in good working order.

4. Alcohol deadens the nerves. When the blood carries alcohol through every part of the body, some of it touches the nerves. In this way it harms the nerves that carry messages to the muscles, and makes them too dull to do their work as they ought. The muscles do not get the right orders from the mind,

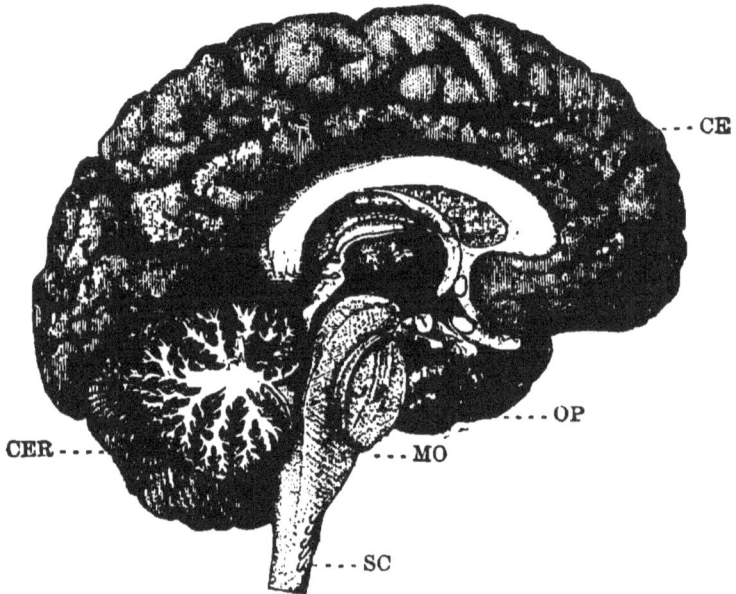

and they do not act as they should. They become weak and trembling.

5. A person who takes wine or cider, or a little brandy or whiskey, may get only a little alcohol, but that little will put his nerves partly to sleep. If he then attempts to do any fine work he cannot do it as well. The nerves that should have guided his muscles exactly are deadened by the alcohol. If he takes more liquor the nerves will be deadened still more. Those that should carry messages to and from the brain will be unable to do so.

6. When a man drinks much liquor he staggers and reels, because he cannot make his muscles do as he wants them to do. He may think very hard about it, and try to make them obey orders, but they cannot. Soon this man will have weak, trembling muscles, even when he is not drunk. His nerves will be so much harmed that they cannot direct the muscles how to move steadily at any time. He will not be able to do work that has to be done by steady hands and a nice touch.

> *Muscles and nerves are stronger without alcohol.*
> *Tobacco harms the nerves and muscles.*

In the next lesson you will learn more about how tobacco harms the nerves, brain, and muscles.

LESSON XII.

MORE ABOUT ALCOHOL, TOBACCO, AND THE BRAIN.

1. But what about the mind itself? Does that remain unharmed while the nerves are being deadened by alcohol? No. Here is the worst condition of all. You have learned that when a person drinks any liquor containing alcohol, this poison quickly passes into the blood and thus is carried to his brain. The way such a person acts shows that the alcohol is affecting the brain more or less, according to the amount that he has drunk. He may talk foolishly, often his good sense seems to have left him, and, worse still, he seems careless about doing right.

2. Just think of the work the brain has to do! It is all the while busy as we study and think, or plan our work or play. The strong, biting alcohol shrivels and hardens the brain so that it can neither think nor plan as well, nor correctly guide the muscles to do their work. By examining the bodies of persons who were killed by drinking, the doctors have found that more of the alcohol goes to the brain than to any other part of the body.

3. Alcohol is a brain poison. When taken day after day it often ruins the brain. A wise English doctor [1] says that "the brain of a person who has been once dead drunk, will never again be so good a brain as it otherwise would have been."

4. One of the worst things about drinking liquor is that it is very apt to make people wicked. It takes away their senses, and then they often do wicked and horrible deeds. It causes some to steal, and others to murder. If you could go into the prisons and ask the prisoners what has brought them there, very many of them would say, "I would not have done the wicked deed that brought me to prison if I had not drunk liquor. It was drink that did it."

5. No one knows when he begins to drink wine or beer or cider, what the alcohol in these drinks will do to him, or make him do. The habit of using alcohol is very easy to form but very hard to break. Some of us may think that we have strong wills and that we can break away from such a habit whenever we choose. Many people whose wills were once as strong as ours thought the same when they began to drink. But the alcohol has made their wills so weak, and the desire for alcoholic drinks so strong, that now they think they cannot let it alone, even though they know it is making drunkards of them. It is the nature of alcohol to make drunkards of those who take it.

6. Many people are made crazy by the use of alcoholic liquors. In some asylums where these people

---

are kept, it has been found that nearly one-half of the crazy people there were made crazy from this cause. Not all of these were drinkers themselves. It often happens that the children of those who drink have weak minds or become crazy as they grow older.

7. You often hear people say, " This child looks like its father," or, that one " like its mother." We get more than our looks from our parents. The children of fathers and mothers who drink alcoholic liquors often get the appetite for such drinks from their parents. An appetite of this kind is easily aroused by only a little liquor, and is very hard to overcome. If we never touch beer, cider, wine, or anything that has alcohol in it, we shall not be in danger of creating or rousing this . dreadful craving for drink that has ruined so many.

8. If everybody could know how much people are hurt every time they take alcoholic drinks, not so many would venture to take the poison, and all would be much better, healthier, and happier.

9. Tobacco, also, weakens the brain and nerves. You may have heard some old smoker say that a pipeful of tobacco or a cigar rested him. Do you know why it made him think this? The poison in the tobacco so benumbed his nerves that they did not . carry the tired feeling to the brain. His muscles were just as tired and needed rest, but he did not feel the weariness.

10. One of the uses of our nerves is to tell us

when we are tired or when we are ill, so that we may rest, or take means to cure ourselves if we are ill. Tobacco weakens the nerves so that they become poor reporters, but it can neither rest us when we are tired nor cure us when we are ill.

11. You have learned that after a muscle has been exercised it needs rest. If it does not have proper rest it grows weak from overwork. This is true of all parts of the body. If we would be well and strong, we must not only take plenty of exercise but we must keep our nerves in good order, so they will tell us when we need rest.

12. The use of tobacco dulls the brain where all the nerves centre. A teacher who taught for many years said, " I have never known a boy who used tobacco to be very bright and thorough in his studies." It is found to be the rule that the boys who have the best standing in their classes at school or college are those who do not use tobacco.

What boy who has a bright mind can afford to lose any of his brightness? This he will be likely to do if he smokes or chews tobacco.

TEST QUESTIONS FOR REVIEW.

THE MUSCLES, BRAIN, AND NERVES.

Lesson IX.—What moves all parts of your body? Tell how the muscles make parts move. How are they fastened to the bones? Do they all move bones? Why do so many end in slender cords? How much of your body is muscle? What will plenty of play and work do for your body?

Lesson X.—What muscles should have exercise? What muscles are strongest? Why is exercise good for the muscles? What does exercise make the heart and lungs do? Why does this do good? When is the best time for exercise? What is said about regular exercise? Tell about the muscles and tight clothing. Why should the muscles have room? What should you not do when you are warm after playing? In what other way can the muscles be injured? What does beer-drinking often do to the muscles? How does fat weaken the muscles? What is said of the health of soldiers who use alcoholic drinks?

Lesson XI.—How does the mind make the muscles work? How do the nerves carry orders? How must the nerves be kept to do their work? What does alcohol do to the nerves? What then happens to the muscles? What makes a drunken man stagger? What will happen to the nerves and muscles, even when such a man is not drunk?

Lesson XII.—What does alcohol do to the brain? What does alcoholic liquor often cause people to do? What does alcohol do to the will? What is it the nature of alcohol to do? How are many people made crazy? What appetite do children sometimes get from parents who drink liquor? How does tobacco treat the nerves? What does it do to the brain? What kind of a mind is the boy who uses tobacco very likely to have?

LESSON XIII.

FOOD: WHY WE NEED IT.

1. Our bodies, like machines that are not alive, wear away by use. Every movement of a bone or a muscle uses up a little of it. Work, play, talking, laughing, and even breathing and thinking, are all the time wearing out particles of our bodies. Strange to tell, some parts of the body are cleaners and pick up worn-out matter that is no longer wanted, and send it out of the body. Now, why is it that your body does not wear away entirely? It is larger, and weighs more than it did a year ago, does it not?

2. The reason is that the body is repaired as fast, sometimes faster, than it wears away. Let us see how this is done. You feel very hungry after you have been playing, don't you? Well, hunger is a sign that your body wants something to put in the place of what has worn out. This something is food. If you are thirsty also, it means water to drink.

3. You want food every few hours, day after day. The more active you are, the more food and water you need. But how do food and drink get to the muscles, bones, and other parts and build them up? You cannot put the food into the muscles and bones. How is it then?

4. Here is the whole story, shortly told. The

things which you eat as food, and the water or milk which you drink, become changed into other things which go to make blood. The blood has in it what will make every part of the body. It is carried all over the body, and when the brain, a nerve, a muscle, or a bone needs anything to strengthen it, it picks out from the blood what it wants. Yes, and it gives up what it no longer wants, and the blood carries it away and sends it out through the lungs, skin, kidneys, etc. In this way the blood is kept pure as well as fresh.

I must eat food that will make bone, muscle, and brain. Exercise gives one a good appetite.

5. How strange it is that all the very different parts of the body are made out of the same building material, — the blood! Our food, if we eat the right kind, contains what is needed to make blood that will do all this.

LESSON XIV.

THE KINDS OF FOOD WE NEED.

1. If a floor wears away, the carpenter uses wood to repair it. If a shoe needs repairing, leather is used. Any article is repaired by using the same kind of material that it was made of. Just so our food, which repairs bone, muscle, brain, and skin, must contain everything that these are made of. It is not safe to depend upon a single kind to do all this, because it may not contain just what is needed. Some articles of food do not contain enough of what the muscles must have, or of what the bones must be repaired with.

2. First let us learn something about foods that make bone and muscle; yes, and other parts as well.

Lean meat, eggs, and vegetable foods, such as the fruits, wheat flour, oat meal, rice, pease, beans, —these all contain matter that the body needs to build it up and make it strong.

3. Now, as you know, many children do not like fat meat. Many eat so much sweet food that it makes them dislike food which is not sweet. This is not right. Fat and sugar are both good foods, but we should not take too much of either of them.

4. Of what use is fatty food? It is very useful in keeping the body warm. Its chief use is to make

heat in the body, and so all people eat it in some
form.   Milk, you know, contains fat,— the fat which
is generally called butter.   Fats are foods that are
like the fatty portions of your body.   In cold weather
we need more fatty food than in warm weather.
People who live in very cold countries eat a great
deal of fat, while those who live in warm countries
eat but little of it.   A little Esquimau boy or girl
is as much pleased when given a pound of tallow
candles to eat, as you are when given a pound of
candy.

We get food from animals,
plants, and minerals.
We must have pure air, pure
water, and proper food.

5. If you chew some grains of wheat, they soon
begin to taste sweet.   This is because the saliva of
your mouth changes the starch in the grains into
sugar.   Starch must be changed into sugar before it
can be made into blood.   In bread, potatoes, oat
meal, and in many vegetables there is starch.   Starch,
like fat, helps to nourish the body and keep it warm.

6. Would you think that there is salt in your blood? You have noticed that the sweat on your skin tastes salty. Well, the sweat comes out from the blood, and so you see that there is salt in your body, and that it is all the time coming out of it. Many of the foods you eat have just a little common salt in them naturaliy, just as your body has. When there is not enough of it in the food we eat, the body soon feels the want of it. The salts in foods go to make bone. All animals need salt. Deer and other animals will travel hundreds of miles in search of it.

7. Well, what are we to learn from all this? Why, that our bodies need both flesh-making foods and heat-making foods; and that it is best to eat a few different articles together. You have heard it said that "too much of one thing is good for nothing," Well, that is quite true of food.

LESSON XV.

HOW THE BLOOD IS MADE.

1. It is very wonderful that blood can be made out of so many different kinds of food as you take into your stomach. Just think of all the different things that you sometimes eat when you have had what you call a good dinner, — turkey, celery, pie, potatoes, grapes, nuts, etc. What a mixture! — and yet red blood can be made out of it. Why, only a few days ago the turkey was strutting about, and now part of him is muscle in your arm! The other articles you ate are also changed as greatly. All now form a part of your body.

2. You have heard people talk about digestion of food. Well, digestion means changing of food into blood. Now let us first notice what is done to the food in the mouth. The mouth is a mill for grinding the food. In it are the teeth to cut and grind, and the finer they grind the better it is. If the teeth are not firm and strong, they cannot do their work well. While they are crushing the food, several little sacs, or *glands*, near the sides of the mouth, pour into it a watery liquid called *saliva.*

It is important to take good care of the teeth.

The stomach has no teeth, and cannot chew food.

3. It takes some time for the saliva to moisten the food and change the starchy part of it into sugar. So you see why it is that you should not swallow the

food too soon, but should let the mill have time to
do the grinding and mixing. Your stomach cannot
do this — it has no teeth.

4. What next is done with the food? We swallow it, and it passes down the food-tube into the

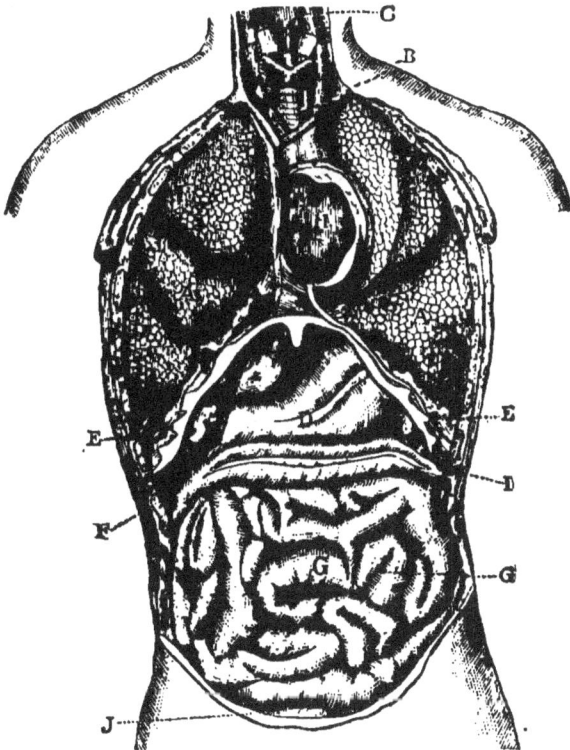

stomach. The stomach is a kind of soft, fleshy bag.
It has a coat of muscles which can make it shrink
and then stretch out larger again. In this way it
moves the food, rolls it around, and mixes it with a
juice which it pours out from its lining. Then, too,

the stomach is warm — as warm as your blood. In this way the busy stomach works away for two to four hours after you have eaten your dinner. At last the food is changed into a thin paste. The warmth, the juice, and the churning have done this. Does the stomach feel tired after its work? It would try to go to work again. But it ought to have rest after hard work. On the preceding page is a picture of the trunk. You can notice how the stomach and bowels are packed away in its lower part. Above you see the heart and lungs in the chest.

5. The lining of the stomach is very thin, thinner than the finest paper, and it is full of tiny blood-vessels. Some of the food has been changed into a fluid which looks like milk, and this soaks through the thin lining into the little blood-vessels. So you see that some of the food gets into the blood in this way. Part of it is not yet ready to go into the blood.

6. Little by little the rest of the food slips out of a small opening in the stomach, and passes into the *bowels.* This is a tube about thirty feet long, but is folded up in the lower room of the trunk in such a way that it is not crowded. Here something else happens to the food. Two other juices pour in upon it and dissolve it still more.

7. As the milky food moves along, more and more of it soaks into the tiny blood-vessels and mixes with the blood. It then becomes a part of the blood and goes on its way to the heart. The heart sends it to all parts of the body. Every little particle of muscle, nerve, and bone is fed by it.

LESSON XVI.

A TALK ABOUT EATING.

1. What a great blessing it is to have good teeth and a healthy stomach! Everybody should try to keep these in good order because good health may be kept by doing so. If the teeth are not kept clean they will decay and be useless. What then? Why, the stomach will have to try to do their work and its own also. This is not fair, for it abuses the stomach. The first thing you should do after eating is to clean the teeth, and in this way keep them sound so that they can chew solid food properly.

2. Now there is something else to think of. Many people take a sip of water, tea, or coffee, with every bit of dry food. This is not a good thing to do. These can moisten the food, but they cannot do what saliva does. Saliva, you know, changes starch in the food into a kind of sugar. So we should eat slowly, and not be in so great a hurry to swallow the food. Let the juice of the mouth do its part. Keep on chewing, and the saliva will moisten the food and make it taste better.

3. What do you think happens when you take a cold drink with your food? Why, the stomach stops work. It was just warm enough before to do its

work, and the cold drink chilled it. It then had to
wait till it became warm again, and this delayed
digestion. In the same way, very cold food stops
digestion for a time. Very hot food does harm also.

4. When the stomach is full after you have eaten,
it presses up against the lungs. This is why it is so
hard to breathe when you run soon after dinner.
It is not well to exercise just after a full meal. Running and playing hard will disturb the stomach. Sit
still for a half-hour, at least. You can study or play
much better afterward.

5. We know a little girl who never has a good
appetite when she comes to the table. She nibbles
a little of one thing and then of another, but she
doesn't want to eat. Why, what is the matter? Well,
her stomach is always tired! She makes it work
most of the time while she is awake. She eats a good
deal of candy between meals. Often she has a piece
of pie or cake — sometimes more than one of each —
before and after meal-time. She doesn't look well,
and she doesn't feel happy.

6. We should eat at regular hours. It is best to
take three meals a day, five or six hours apart. This
will give the stomach time to digest the food, and to
rest a while afterwards. It will then be ready for
more food when meal-time comes again.

7. It is easy to tell when too much food is taken.
Too much food makes us feel uncomfortable, and
sometimes causes pain. If we eat a full meal just
before going to bed, we may not sleep well, but be

restless and have bad dreams. Such sleep does not rest the body and the brain.

> *Children should not take a meal when they are heated and excited by play.*

8. Don't eat unwholesome food. Hot and moist bread is not good food. It gives the stomach hard work. Unripe fruit is unwholesome. Pie, cake, and candy are unwholesome when they are eaten freely, like bread and fruit. It is very foolish to overload the stomach with what we do not need, just because it tastes good. We should not allow dainties to tempt us to eat more than we need. And we should never flavor our pies, puddings, or other food with wine or brandy, for fear we shall come to like the taste of alcohol if we use it in this way.

If we are not wise about our eating, we shall give the whole body a great deal of trouble. If our food is not digested well, we cannot be strong, healthy, and happy.

LESSON XVII.

DRINKS: WATER, TEA, AND COFFEE.

1. We use water so often as a drink that we seldom think how good and refreshing it is. Once in a while we happen to be very thirsty, and then we think of this. If we are parched with fever, we think of sparkling, cold water as the very best thing in all the world.

You may have heard of people escaping in boats from a sinking ship, and of how terribly they suffered from thirst. Briny water all around them, but not a drop of it fit to be drunk! Fresh water was almost the only thing they could think of. One after another sank down, moaning and dying from thirst.

2. We can live longer without food than without water. Why is it? Well, you may be surprised to learn that about three-fourths of your body is made up of water. It is everywhere in our bodies. The blood could not flow in the arteries and veins if there was not a great deal of water in it. The water makes it flow along easily. A great deal of water is all the time leaving our bodies, and taking along with it waste matter that we are well rid of. Every breath sends out watery vapor from the lungs. Sweat is constantly passing out through the skin, and the kidneys also take water from the blood.

3. Now you can see that there must be some way to make up for the loss. How do we know when to take in water? Why, we feel thirsty, and that means that the blood is asking for water and must have it. Milk, you know, quenches thirst because there is so much water in it. Yes, and it is excellent food as well.

Of course we take a great deal of water in moist food, such as ripe fruit, vegetables, lean meat, fish, etc. But when we are very thirsty, nothing else is quite so good as clear water.

Of all drinks, pure water is the best.

Alcoholic drinks cannot quench thirst; they make thirst.

4. People are learning to be more careful about the kind of water they drink. Even when water seems clean, there may be something in it that would cause dreadful sickness. Many deaths have been caused by drinking impure water. Water that runs through lead pipes may have a little lead dissolved in it, and lead is poisonous. It is safest to let water run a little while from such pipes before you drink it.

5. Have you seen a well in a barnyard, or near a pig-pen or other filthy place? It may be that slops also are thrown on the ground near it. Now the filthy things about such a well sink down through the ground and get into the water. Of course the water is not fit for drinking or cooking. A short time since the people of a whole village were poisoned by drinking water from a stream into which slops from a sick-room had run. Many of the people died of fever.

6. Some children drink *tea* and *coffee.* Perhaps your parents do not allow you to do so. Well, that is right. Tea and coffee are not good for children. There is something in both of these drinks that does harm to young bodies. Many grown people find that tea and coffee injure their stomachs, make them nervous, and cause headache. You do not need tea and coffee, and so it is much better to drink wholesome milk and pure water. Milk with hot water in it makes a nice, warm drink. It gives warmth and comfort without doing harm.

LESSON XVIII.

WHAT ALCOHOL AND TOBACCO DO TO THE STOMACH.

1. You have been told about a peculiar juice which pours in upon the food in the stomach. This is the *gastric juice.* Without it the food could not be dissolved. If you take anything into your stomach which is strong enough to spoil or weaken the gastric juice, digestion will have to stop. Alcohol is just such a dangerous thing. It cannot dissolve the food itself, while it so changes the gastric juice that it cannot dissolve the food as it otherwise would.

2. Few people drink clear alcohol. It is too strong to be drunk in that state. It would destroy the lining of the mouth, throat, and stomach at once. The strongest drinks are about one-half alcohol, and these are so strong that they burn the mouth. Cider, beer, wine, gin, rum, and whiskey are the usual forms in which alcohol is drunk. A drop of brandy put into your eye would make it smart and look red. Alcoholic drinks do the same to the inside of the stomach. They often make inflamed and sore stomachs.

3. Now you can see that if these alcoholic liquors can spoil the gastric juice and do so much harm to the stomach, no one should drink them. A diseased stomach cannot change food into good blood. Such a stomach does not call for food, but for more strong drink to quiet its bad feelings for a little while, and the more the drinker takes, the worse off his stomach is.

4. If you know that anything you eat hurts you and makes you ill, you do not eat it again. Now we have learned beforehand that alcohol will injure us; and so, if we are wise, we shall not give it a chance to harm us even once.

We should not take any-thing into the stomach that will do it harm.

It is very easy to get into a habit of using alcohol and tobacco.

5. You see that the stomach is a kind of kitchen in the body. If things go wrong in the kitchen, there is trouble in the whole house. If the cook in the kitchen takes strong drink, the dinner is apt to be spoiled.

6. Do you know some boys who have begun to use tobacco? They only smoke cigarettes! But these are made of tobacco, and tobacco is very poisonous. The very poorest kind is often used in cigarettes. There is very good reason to believe that very many boys die every year from cigarette-smoking. They may appear to get used to it, and you may not see that it does them harm. You know that it made them deathly sick at first. Well, that is not the least of the harm it does.

7. How does tobacco do harm? In several ways. Some of the poison juice gets into the stomach and makes it weak. This causes dyspepsia. It spoils the appetite for food, and then the body becomes weak. It poisons the blood, and makes it less able to nourish the body. So you can easily see that it prepares the body for disease. It gives weakness, not strength.

Boys, if you would have strong muscles and nerves, bright minds, sound hearts, and pure blood, don't learn to smoke tobacco.

TEST QUESTIONS FOR REVIEW.

FOOD AND DIGESTION.

Lesson XIII. — What things cause our bodies to wear away? Why does not your body wear away entirely? What is hunger a sign of? What does your body need every few hours? How is the food you eat changed? What does it make? What has the blood in it? Where does the blood go, and what does it do? What do the parts of your body do with the things they no longer want? What keeps the blood pure and fresh?

Lesson XIV. — What must be in the food we eat? Why? Why is it not best to take only one kind of food? Why must we eat such food? Why should you not eat too much sweet food? Are sugar and fat good foods? Of what use is fatty food? When do we need more fatty food? What articles of food have starch in them? Is starchy food good for your body? Why? How do you know that there is salt in your blood? Tell what you read about the need of salt. What two great kinds of food do we need? What is said about eating different articles together?

Lesson XV. — What does digestion mean? What is done to food in the mouth? What if the teeth are not firm and strong? Tell about the saliva and what it does. Why should you not swallow the food too soon? What next is done to the food? Tell what the stomach does to the food. How long does it take the stomach to change the food? Does the stomach grow tired? How does the food get into the blood from the stomach? Where does some of the food go from the stomach? What happens to the food after it goes into the bowels? At last where does the food go with the blood, and where is it sent?

Lesson XVI. — Why should you take care of your teeth? When should you brush them? Why is it not best to take drink with every mouthful of dry food? What will moisten the food in the mouth? Tell what harm it does to take cold drink with your food. Tell what is said about very cold or very hot food. Why should you not run or play hard just after a meal? What is best to do then? Tell what is said about the little girl who never has an appetite for her meals. When and how often should we eat? Why? How can we know when we have eaten too much? What is said about eating just before we go to bed? Mention some kinds of food that are unwholesome. What is said about eating pie, cake, and candy? About dainties? What harm will come if we are not careful about our eating?

Lesson XVII. — Which can we do without longer, food or water? How much of your body is water? Of what use is water in our bodies? What is all the time becoming of the water in our bodies? How do we make up for its loss? How do we know when the body needs water? What kinds of food contain a good deal of water? What is the best of all drinks? What kind of water is harmful? Tell what is said about water that runs through lead pipes. How do barnyards, pig-pens, and slops make water bad in wells? Are tea and coffee good drinks for children? Why not? What drinks are much better for you?

Lesson XVIII. — What is the name of the juice that changes the food in the stomach? What if you drink anything that will spoil this juice? What does alcohol do to the gastric juice? What would happen if any one should drink clear alcohol? How much alcohol is there in the strongest drinks? How do such strong drinks hurt the stomach? What if the stomach is harmed and its juice is spoiled? When we know that alcohol will harm us, what should we do? What harm does smoking tobacco do to the stomach? To the appetite? To the blood? If you want strong muscles and bright minds, what must you let alone? Who are harmed greatly by tobacco?

LESSON XIX.

THE HEART : HOW THE BLOOD MOVES.

1. In a tree the sap goes up in one set of pipes, and goes down in another set. Just so the blood in your body is always in motion. There are two sets of pipes for it to go back and forth in; these two sets are called *arteries* and *veins*. It used to be thought that the blood moved backward and forward in the same tubes.

2. The blood in your body is kept in motion by a strawberry-shaped pump about as large as your fist. This little pump is your heart. Night and day, never stopping to rest, it beats away as long as you live. If it is healthy, it beats regularly, and not by fits and starts. That, you know, is the right way to do all work.

3. If you could look into your heart, what do you think you would see? Why, it is hollow; or, rather, there are four rooms in it, two above and two below. What strange little rooms they are, full of blood! Yes, and see how their walls move in and out! When the walls draw inward, the blood is squeezed out into a large tube. From this great

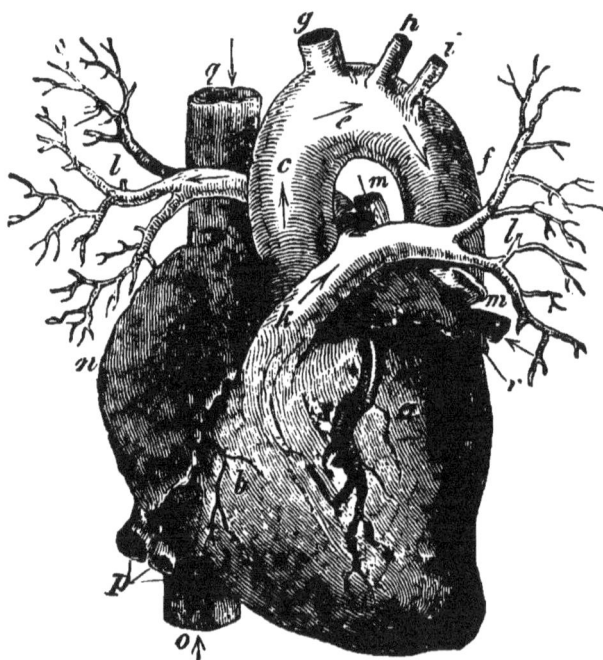

main tube other tubes branch out everywhere, and carry the nourishing blood to all parts of the body. The smallest tubes are finer than the finest hair. The blood in these little tubes makes the lips red.

Above is a picture of the heart. In it you see the great main blood-vessels, marked *c*, whose branches carry the blood to all parts of your body. The lungs have been taken away, but you can see the blood-vessels that go into them branching out like the limbs and twigs of trees.

4. The heart keeps on pumping, and at last the blood turns back, through another set of tubes, toward the heart. It has made a journey of the whole body, and now it flows back by two large tubes into one of the rooms of the heart.

5. The blood goes out of the heart by the arteries; it comes back by the veins. When it goes out, it is bright red; when it comes back it is dark and filled with impure particles. It is then sent into the lungs to be made pure by the fresh air.

Pure air helps to make pure blood.

Alcohol and tobacco weaken the heart.

6. You can see that if the heart should stop pump ing, the body would die. Anything that interferes with the work of the heart does harm. The blood must move properly to keep the body healthy.

7. Every time the heart squeezes the blood out, it moves forward a little and knocks against the ribs. This knocking can be felt plainly after you exercise because the heart beats more quickly then. If you suddenly become very angry, the heart seems to know it, because it makes a great jump. If it is not strong, this may do great harm. People have died from a fit of anger.

8. You can see some of the veins just under the skin. The dark blood in them makes them appear blue. You cannot see the arteries, because they nearly all lie deep. Suppose you were to tie a cord tightly round your arm near the shoulder. What would happen? The arm would become pale and begin to grow cold. It would seem to grow very heavy and clumsy, and after a while the feeling in it would be altogether lost. What has the tight cord done? Why, it has pressed on the arteries and veins so as to stop the blood from moving in them.

9. What if you wear a tight collar? Of course it will press upon the blood-vessels in the neck and keep the blood from moving back and forth. This may cause headache and fainting. Tight garters, tight sleeves, and tight clothing of any kind keep the blood from moving freely and do great harm. Think how cold and painful our hands and feet are if we wear tight gloves and tight shoes. All these things make hard work for the heart.

LESSON XX.

HOW ALCOHOL AND TOBACCO INJURE THE HEART AND BLOOD-VESSELS.

1. You would think it very cruel to whip a good horse who is willing and is going fast enough. You would not abuse such a horse. Now let us see how it is with the heart. It is made of muscle, and is always doing just about as much work as it should do. But what do you think happens when the alcohol that has been taken into the blood reaches the heart? Why, just as a spur stuck into a horse makes him go faster, so the alcohol seems to spur the heart and make it work faster.

2. Now all this hard work is useless; it is strength thrown away. This extra work makes the heart tired and weak. After the alcohol goes away, the heart cannot work as quickly as it did before the alcohol was taken. It is not able to do its regular work, and it takes some time to get back its strength.

3. Worse than all, when alcohol is constantly used, it may slowly change the muscles of the heart into fat. Such a heart cannot be as strong as if it were all muscle. It is sometimes so soft that a finger could easily be pushed through its walls. You can think what may happen if it is made to work a little harder than usual. It is liable to stretch and stop beating, and this would cause sudden death.

4. Let us see what this same alcohol may do to the blood-vessels, for it passes through them as well. When it touches the nerves that control the blood-vessels, it .deadens them and makes them so weak that they lose their grip. The blood-vessels then become limp, and more blood flows into them and swells them out. You can see how this looks in the red, blotched face of a hard drinker. It is just so in his brain, and in his lungs and stomach.

5. After a while alcohol is apt to make the blood-vessels hard and brittle. What then? Why, they may break when the blood is pumped hard into them. If one in the brain bursts, the blood flows out and is very apt to cause death. So you see that alcohol is a great trouble-maker everywhere in the body.

6. *Tobacco* also injures the heart. It sometimes fattens and weakens it, and makes it work badly. Very many who use tobacco have unsteady hearts. Have you not heard it said that some one had a *"tobacco heart"*? That means that the heart had been put out of order by smoking or chewing tobacco. You have already been told how it poisons the blood and makes trembling nerves ; yes, and that it spoils appetite for food and makes the stomach weak.

7. You can understand that if the blood is to feed all the parts of the body, and build them up, it must be good blood. Anything that gets into the blood and changes it from its good condition is sure to do harm everywhere. Both alcohol and tobacco make such changes in the blood and spoil it. Sometimes they make the blood too thick; again, too thin. We may say, then, that both alcohol and tobacco poison the blood. When the blood is poisoned by them, the brain becomes diseased, the nerves are weakened, and the person may become crazy.

———•◦•———

TEST QUESTIONS FOR REVIEW.

THE BLOOD.

Lesson XIX. — Tell about the two sets of pipes in which your blood moves. What are they called? What keeps your blood in motion? How does the heart work when it is healthy? Tell about the rooms of the heart. How does the blood get out of the heart? Tell about the tubes that go out from it. How does the blood get back to the heart? What kind of blood goes out from the heart? What kind comes back to it? Where is the impure blood then sent? What if the heart should stop working? Tell about the beating of the heart. What does it do when you become suddenly angry? What harm may this do? What if anything is tied tightly about your arm? What if you wear tight clothing? Mention some things that keep the blood from moving.

Lesson XX. — Of what is the heart made? When alcohol gets to the heart, what does it make it do? How does the heart feel after the alcohol goes away? How can alcohol change the heart? What may happen when the heart is made fat? What harm does alcohol do to the blood-vessels and nerves in them? What if the blood-vessels break? What harm does tobacco do to the heart? What is said of the hearts of many who use tobacco? How do alcohol and tobacco spoil the blood?

LESSON XXI.

THE AIR WE BREATHE: BAD AIR.

1. You cannot see air, and yet it is something. You cannot feel it when it is not moving, as you can water. If you fan yourself the air is moved, and you can feel it strike against your face. When the wind blows hard you can feel the air push and strike hard against you, and you can see how it makes the great trees bend and shake.

2. Air is a kind of food for plants and animals. They could not live without it. We do not eat or drink it, and so we do not take it into our bodies as we do food and water that go down into the stomach. We breathe it into our lungs, and it is necessary to our lives. If it were shut out from our lungs, even for a few minutes, we should die. There is a pure gas, called *oxygen,* in the air that makes the blood pure and gives it life.

3. Now let us see how the air reaches the blood. When the blood comes back in the veins to the heart, it is dark and is not good blood. It has been everywhere in the body, and the muscles, bones, nerves, and skin have all taken out of it what they need. It is not fit to be sent back to them again as long as it is dark, impure blood. It must get the new blood that has been made out of the food, and it must in

some way be changed into good, red blood. Now
the place where this is done is the lungs.

4. Hear is a picture of the heart and lungs, which,
you know, fill up your chest. The lungs are marked
a and *b*, and they are drawn aside so that you can
see the heart which is marked *d*. The wind-pipe is
marked *c*, and the air goes down through it into the
lungs. The lungs are light and spongy because they
are full of tiny air-sacks.

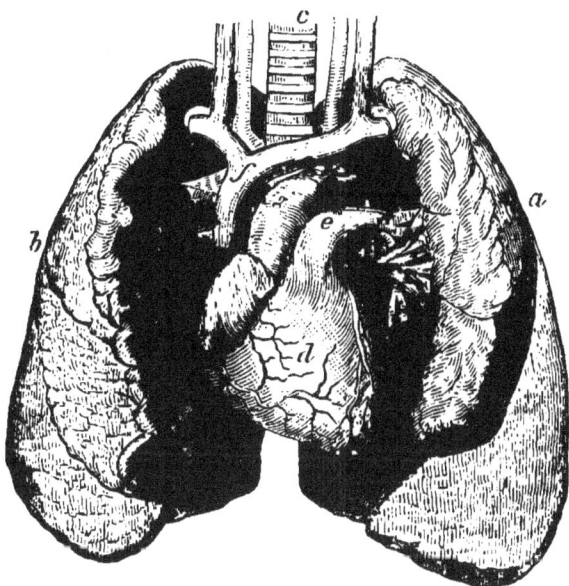

5. Every time you breathe, the air goes down
into the little air-bags in the lungs. Now there is
only a very thin skin between the air in the little
sacks and the tiny blood-vessels in the lungs, and so
the sacks are not perfectly air-tight. Air gets in

through the thin skin to the blood it finds in the little vessels, and changes it to a bright red.

6. But while the blood in the lungs is taking in air, it is also sending out worn-out matter that is no longer needed, and a poisonous gas that got into the blood as it went about the body. When you breathe out, these waste matters pass out from your lungs in your breath.

7. Now you can see why it is that you have to breathe to keep alive. Yes, and you can understand that the air which has been once in your lungs should not be taken in again. It is worn-out air, and is poisonous and unfit to go back into the lungs. It cannot make pure blood, but it can cause disease.

8. A mouse was once put into a glass jar, where no air could either get out or in. It soon became very restless. It panted and breathed hard. After a little while it fell over senseless and died. It could not get fresh air, and so had to breathe over and over the bad air that had been in its lungs. Just so it would be with us if we were kept in a small, close room, and could not let fresh air come in. The air in such a room soon becomes very bad, and we begin to breathe hard, grow faint, and would die in a short time.

9. Yes, we must have fresh air to breathe as well as wholesome food to eat and pure water to drink. And we need pure air every moment, day and night. The air in your school-room soon grows bad because there are so many to breathe it. Unless fresh air is

let in, you breathe the poisonous air over and over.
This makes you feel dull and tired because you have
used up so much of the good air, and have begun·to
breathe the poisonous gas you have just read about.

10. You know that we pass many hours in our
sleeping-room. Yes, about one-third of our lives.
Well, you can see that we should be very careful to
let fresh air come into our bed-rooms, else we shall
breathe bad air most of this time. It may be that
you have noticed the unpleasant smell of a close
room, or of a bed-room that had been tightly closed
all night. Do you wonder that people do not feel
rested, and that they have headache and lose appetite, when they breathe such bad air?

11. We should let pure air come into our rooms
by night as well as by day. If we have plenty of
clothes on our beds, we shall not feel too cold if a
window is left open an inch or two at the top, even
in winter. We can manage it so that the air shall
not blow upon us and give us colds.

LESSON XXII.

HOW TO BREATHE.

1. "How· to breathe! Why, who does not know
how to breathe?" you ask. Well, let us see how
that is. We should take in enough air at each breath
to fill our lungs, else they will not have as much air

as is needed to purify the blood. If we do not draw in enough air at each breath, we must breathe faster, and this tires the muscles.

2. Now, many people only partly fill their lungs at each of the short breaths they take. They breathe so quickly that the air is sent out again before it can do its work. Many get this wrong habit from standing and sitting in bad positions, and from tight clothing about the chest. You should keep good positions in standing and sitting, and should try to have your clothing so loose that it will not press upon the chest and hinder full breathing.

3. Can we train ourselves to breathe properly? Certainly we can. Here is a good exercise in breathing for children: Stand erect, arms and shoulders thrown back, and toes turned out. Now breathe in slowly enough air to fill your lungs. When they are full, beat your chest moderately with your closed hands, and then let the air out slowly. Fill your lungs slowly again, and this time strike out with your fists, upward, downward, and straight ahead. You should repeat this exercise every day in the open air, or in a room with the window open.

4. You should not get a habit of breathing through your mouth. The nose is the true breathing-passage, and the air gets warmed in passing through it. When we breathe through the mouth, a large stream of cold, dry air reaches the throat and lungs. You know how dry the mouth and throat get when you run and breathe through the mouth. Well, people who breathe through the mouth all the time are more apt to get sore throats and sore lungs. You know how silly the open mouth makes the face look. Awake or asleep, we should breathe through the nose.

5. Many children cover their heads with the blankets and fall asleep in that way. This is a harmful habit, because the air under the bed-clothes soon becomes bad and is breathed over and over. This bad habit has been known to make children pale and unhealthy.

Use your voice but little when your throat or lungs are sore.

Filth or slops poison the air.

When air smells bad there is danger in it.

We should try to keep the air of our rooms pure, and to breathe it in the right way.

LESSON XXIII.

EFFECTS OF ALCOHOL AND TOBACCO UPON THE AIR-PASSAGES.

1. Every part of the body to which alcohol goes in the blood seems anxious to get rid of it. The stomach cannot change it because it is not food, and so hurries it out, just as it is, into the blood. It soon goes to the heart, and the heart hurries it off to the lungs, and they send some of it out in the breath. Some of it is sent out by the kidneys, and the skin also sends it out in the sweat.

2. If a man drinks a good deal of alcohol, it may take a day, or longer, to get rid of it. You can easily notice how a drinker smells of alcohol when you come near him. All this time the alcohol is doing the mischief; and when it comes out in the breath from the lungs, or in the sweat from the skin, it is alcohol yet. The body has not been able to make any good use of it at all.

3. But let us see what alcohol does when it goes with the blood into the lungs. You have just read about the delicate air-cells in the lungs, and that they are made of the finest kind of skin. Now, when the alcohol touches the air-cells, it thickens the delicate skin, and so makes it hard for air to pass through into the blood. Besides, you can see that waste matter from the blood finds it just as hard to pass out.

4. Now, in these ways alcohol does mischief in the lungs. It keeps the blood from being made pure, when people drink much of it. You know that a cold when it settles upon the lungs is very dangerous. When the lungs are injured by drinking liquor, a cold is apt to be a very serious thing, and is very hard to cure. Many drinkers die at such a time. Lungs irritated by alcohol are not in good condition to bear up against a cold. The thickened lining of the lungs makes the breathing-space too small.

5. Other air-passages are irritated by alcohol. No doubt you have heard the hoarse, wheezy voice of a man who drinks a great deal of liquor. The lining skin of his throat is thickened and dried, and so his voice is broken and husky. You feel as though clearing your throat would help him to use his voice more easily. Now let us see what harm tobacco does.

6. Tobacco smoke has in it many fine particles that are breathed in and lodge in the air-passages and lungs. This irritates the lining of the nose, throat and lungs, and does much harm. Irritation of the air-passages of the nose and throat leads to catarrh. Tobacco smoking may cause consumption by making diseased lungs. It also benumbs the nerves of taste and smell. The sense of taste sometimes is so blunted by tobacco that plain food is tasteless: those who use tobacco are apt to take strongly peppered and spiced food to wake up the sense of taste. This does harm to the stomach.

7. It is well known that tobacco injures the voice. We hear the husky voices of many people who smoke or chew a great deal of the poisonous weed. Many good singers would not think for a moment of using tobacco in any form. Cigarettes are especially harmful, because much of the smoke gets into the air-passages and inflames them. The burning paper makes them still more harmful. Surely, it is a silly habit to smoke or chew tobacco!

TEST QUESTIONS FOR REVIEW.

AIR AND BREATHING.

Lesson XXI.—Of what use is air to plants and animals? How do we take it into our bodies? What is there in air to make the blood pure? What kind of blood comes back to the heart from the body? Tell about the lungs. How does air get into the blood in the lungs? What does the impure blood give up? Why should you not breathe the same air over again? What harm will bad air do? Tell about the mouse in the tight jar. What if you were kept in an air-tight room? What is said about having good air in your school-room? Tell what you read about keeping good air in your bed-room. How may it be managed safely?

Lesson XXII.—How much air should you take at each breath? Why? In what wrong way do many people breathe? What causes them to do so? What is said about keeping good positions and loose clothing? Tell about the good breathing exercise. Why should you not breathe through your mouth? What did you read about sleeping with your head covered with the blankets?

Lesson XXIII.—What does the body try to do with the alcohol taken into it? What does the stomach do with it? The heart? The lungs? The skin? What is alcohol doing while it stays in the body? Can the body make good use of it? What harm does alcohol do to the lungs? What harm does it do to the blood? Tell about the danger of a cold when the lungs are harmed by alcohol: Tell what alcohol may do to the voice. How does tobacco smoke injure the air-passages and lungs? What does tobacco do to the nerves of taste and smell? Why are cigarettes particularly harmful?

LESSON XXIV.

THE SKIN AND ITS WORK: BATHING.

1. How snugly the skin fits our bodies, and yet it is so elastic that it is not too tight! It protects the tender flesh, helps to keep the body warm, and lets out waste matter from the blood. Yes, and it has been found out that it takes in air and gives out a gas like that which the lungs send out. To do its work well, the skin must be cared for. It must be washed and kept clean.

2. Perhaps you have never thought that you have two skins. Well, you really have two. First, there is a thin layer on the outside, and this is called the *scarf skin*. It is constantly wearing away, and drops off in fine powder or little scales. It washes off when you take a bath. It has neither blood-vessels nor nerves, and cutting it does not draw blood nor cause pain. In a blister, water gathers under this outer skin and puffs it up.

3. Under the scarf skin there is a thicker one, called the *true skin*. It is full of little blood-vessels and nerves. If a needle pricks down to this inner skin, it draws blood, and you feel it very quickly because it touches the nerves.

4. When the outer skin is scraped off by a fall, you can see the red, inner skin. It stings and pains when it is uncovered, because the nerves cannot even bear to have the air touch them. So you can see that the outer skin takes care of the nerves, and keeps things from touching them or rubbing against them. The nerves can feel well enough through the outer skin, because it is so thin. You know how easily the nerves in the tips of your fingers can feel anything that touches the skin on them.

5. Look at the tips of your fingers and see the curved ridges in the skin. Now if you look at these ridges through a strong microscope, you will see that they are full of little holes. It is the same in the skin all over the body. There are millions of them altogether. They are called *pores*, and are the mouths of little tubes that run out from the inner skin. The sweat is constantly getting into these little tubes from the blood, and they pour it out upon the outer skin. Salt and worn-out particles float out in the sweat. About a pint of it passes out of the blood every day.

6. When we are very warm, the sweat pours out faster than it dries, and we see it. At other times it dries as fast as it comes out. But there are also other little tubes that pour out a kind of oil, to keep the skin soft and the hair glossy. Sometimes this oil gets hardened in the little tubes, and little bits of dirt get into the outer ends of them. When this is squeezed out, it looks like a little white worm with a black head.

7. What do you think would happen if your skin were varnished over with something that would stop up the mouths of all these little tubes? Death would happen very soon. A little boy was once covered with gold gilt, so as to look like a cherub. He became ill very soon after the performance. In spite of all that was done he died in a few hours, because the gilt and varnish were not washed from his skin.

8. Now, when the sweat and oil come out upon the skin, they get mixed with the loose, powdery scales of the outer skin. When this is not often washed off, it dries into a kind of pasty varnish, and stops up the mouths of the sweat-tubes and oil-tubes. This keeps them from doing their work as they should do it. The skin should be kept free from such a dirty varnish.

Try to have clean, dry cloth= ing next to the skin.

9. How often should you wash the whole body? A bath every day is a good thing for most peo-

ple. You should wash the whole skin at least twice
a week in winter, and oftener in summer. Always
give the skin a good rubbing to dry and warm it
after a bath. Bathing in cool water makes the skin
active and healthy.

10. Here are a few good cautions about bathing :
Don't bathe in cold water when you are warm after
play. Get cool first. Don't stay in the water till
you feel chilly, for it is dangerous to do so. Come
out before you begin to feel cold. You should not
take a bath just after a full meal. Wait for an
hour or two. Don't sit down where the air blows
upon you after a bath, for you may take cold in that
way. If you are chilly, take exercise. Don't go into
deep water until you can swim very well. You cannot be too careful while learning to swim.

LESSON XXV.

HOW ALCOHOL AND TOBACCO HARM THE SKIN.

1. What a beautiful, soft covering for the body a
healthy skin makes! No face can be quite pretty
when the skin is not healthy. The blood must be
pure and must move properly to keep the skin
healthy. Now you have been told that wholesome
food, plenty of exercise and fresh air, and washing
the body often, keep the blood in good order. You

must try to take all of these if you wish to have an active, beautiful skin.·

2. The skin has a great deal of work to do, and our bodies cannot be very healthy if we let anything harm the skin. You see how red and harsh-looking alcohol makes the faces of people who drink much of it.

3. You remember that alcohol deadens the nerves in the walls of the blood-vessels, that should keep these vessels from stretching, and from letting too much blood in. Thus the little blood-vessels are too much crowded with blood, and they shine through the skin and make it look fiery. Sometimes most of the blood of the face seems to get into the skin of the nose. All the little veins look as though they might burst, and blotches and pimples begin to be seen.

4. At first, alcohol makes the skin feel very warm because it drives so much blood into it. But this does not last long. You can see that so much blood sent out so near the air must get cool very soon.

Yes, it does so, and before long the whole body grows colder than it should be. In this way alcohol makes the body so cold that it may freeze to death sooner than without it. Men who travel in the cold parts of the world have found out that they are warmer without drinking brandy, whiskey, or rum. So you can see that alcohol prevents the skin from keeping the body warm.

5. When a boy begins to use tobacco, he often

becomes pale and has an unhealthy skin. Why is this so? Because such a boy weakens his muscles and nerves by using tobacco, and so does not feel like taking exercise. His blood does not move as it should, and this makes his skin pale. This is a sure sign of the harm that tobacco is doing. The skin tells very soon when anything is going wrong in the body.

6. Here is something to think of, boys. A boy who uses tobacco is doing harm to his mind. He cannot study as well as others can who do not use it. He is not apt to keep up with his class, because he is losing strength and feels dull. This makes him hate study and work. Yes, he even hates to play. His mind and body both feel weak from the poison tobacco. If he does not let it alone it may shorten his life many years.

Alcohol and tobacco injure all the senses.

7. Suppose that you were trying to build up something and that some mischievous boy pulled it down as fast as you built it up. Why, you would be much provoked. You would try to make the mischief-maker stop. Well, when you build up your body with good food, pure air, and exercise, and by keeping your skin clean, alcohol and tobacco will spoil all the good that these do, if you let them in. They often go together, like bad boys, to do mischief.

TEST QUESTIONS FOR REVIEW.

THE SKIN AND ITS CARE.

Lesson XXIV.—In what way is your skin useful to your body? How must it be cared for in order to do its work? Tell about your two skins. What is all the time happening to the outer skin? In which skin are the nerves and blood-vessels? Of what use is the outer skin? What are the pores of the skin? Tell about the sweat. Tell about the oil-tubes and what they pour out. What if your skin were varnished with something that would close the pores? Tell about the little boy whose skin was gilded. What happens when sweat, oil, and worn-out skin are not washed off? How often should your body be washed? Why should your skin be rubbed after a bath? Tell what cautions you read about bathing and swimming.

Lesson XXV.—What is said about the blood and a healthy skin? Why is the skin so important to good health? How does alcohol make the skin look? Why is this so? At first how does alcohol make the skin feel? Does it keep the body warm? Why not? Tell about alcohol and death by freezing. What is said about the skin of a boy who uses tobacco? Why does not such a boy like to exercise his body? Tell what is said about the movement of his blood. What is a certain sign of the harm tobacco does him? Tell how it interferes with his studies. What makes him hate study, work, and play? What may tobacco do if the boy does not let it alone? Tell how alcohol and tobacco are like bad boys who do mischief.

LESSON XXVI.

CARE OF EYESIGHT AND HEARING.

1. You are not old enough yet to understand all about the parts of your eyes. You can notice how well they are guarded. They are set in deep, bony sockets, and there are bones all around them except in front. A blow is likely to strike upon some of these bones and not upon the eye itself. In this way it is kept from harm.

2. How quickly the lids close to shut out anything that might touch the eye, and how the tears flow to wash away anything that happens to get into it! In this picture you can see the little sack, marked *a*, that makes the tears. It is in the bony rim above the eye. Little tubes carry the tears from it into the eye. Some of the tears run out into a tube that takes them into the nose.

3. Light gets into the eye through a little round window in the front of it. This little window looks like a round, dark spot. It has a beautiful screen which closes to shut out some of the light when it is too bright, and then the little window looks smaller. But when the light is dim, or in the dark, the screen draws away and lets in all the light it can. The light goes to a nerve in the back of the eye, and this nerve in some way tells the brain, and it sees.

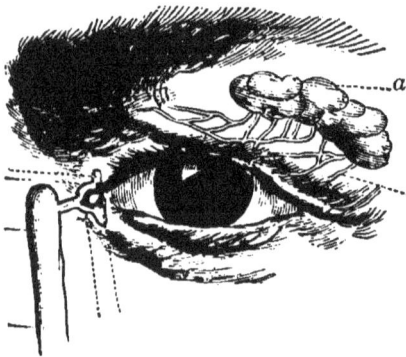

4. When eyes are good, they can see things both near by and far away. Old people often cannot see things that are near their eyes as well as they can see those that are farther away. Many children are near-sighted. That is, they cannot see things very well unless they can bring them close to their eyes. Such children should wear glasses.

5. You can learn to use your eyes properly, and to take such good care of them that they may not grow weak or near-sighted. You all want to keep good eyes, and so you should remember and practise these rules: Do not hold your book too near to your eyes. Don't read or do fine work when the light is dim. Wait till the lamps are lighted. Don't face the light, but let it come from the left or from above you. Don't stoop over your book or work. Don't read while lying down. Stop reading if your eyes smart or feel tired, and let them rest. Keep your slate clean, and make large, plain letters and figures.

6. We need to have good ears as well as good eyes. You have just read how your eyes are guarded. Your ears are also well guarded by bones. The inner parts, where the hearing is done, are in the solid bone of the skull. A tube leads from the outside to the inner parts, and this tube is closed at its inner end by a tight skin, like the head of a drum. Indeed, it is called the drum-head.

7. In the tube of the ear there is a very bitter wax. It keeps the lining moist and soft. Why is it that insects do not often crawl into your ears? They do not like the bitter wax. If one happens to go in, it soon gets covered with the sticky wax, and so cannot do much harm. It soon dies.

8. Children sometimes try to scrape the wax from

their ears with pins, bits of wood, or with the end of
a pencil. They should not do so, for such scraping
things harm the ears, and may burst the drum-head
and cause deafness. It is usually best to let the wax
alone, for it will roll out when it is no longer needed.

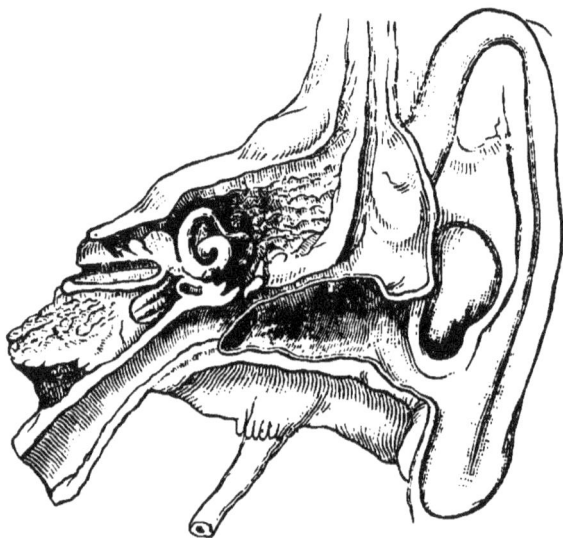

9. If anything gets wedged fast in the tube of
your ear, don't pick at it, for you may push it further
in. It cannot get into your brain unless you push it
through the drum-head. Let it alone, and wait as
patiently as you can till it can be taken out by some
one who knows how to do so safely. Shouting loudly
into any one's ear is a bad, dangerous trick. It
gives the nerves a great shock, and may injure the
hearing.

LESSON XXVII.

ALCOHOL AND TOBACCO INJURE SIGHT AND HEARING.

1. Would you think that drinking liquor and using tobacco could harm eyesight and hearing? They do. Alcohol and tobacco often inflame the eyes. People who drink liquor often have inflamed, blood-shot eyes; and tobacco smoke acts to inflame the eyes, particularly the delicate lining of the lids. You can see, then, that the short cigarettes, burning and smoking so near the face, must be particularly hurtful to the eyes.

2. Besides, both alcohol and tobacco injure the nerves, and so must injure sight in this way also. Those who use much alcohol or tobacco often have poor eyesight. You should think of your eyes as two very precious jewels carefully placed away in a nicely made case, and should be very watchful to keep them from all harm.

3. Now let us see how good hearing may be injured by alcohol and tobacco. Alcohol, you know, is a very hot, biting liquid. Pure alcohol would burn the skin from your mouth and throat. Brandy, whiskey, and the other strong liquors have enough alcohol in them to inflame the throat. Well, in the back part of the throat are the mouths of two little tubes, one going to each ear. Now when the throat gets inflamed by the fiery liquor or strong tobacco smoke, the little tubes also become dry and swollen. If they become closed, or even partly so, hearing is made dull.

LESSON XXVIII.

WHAT TO DO AND WHAT NOT TO DO.

1. Our teeth should be cleansed after every meal. To do this well, place the points of the upper and the lower front teeth together, and then brush up and down. Take good care of the back teeth, for they need even more brushing than the front ones. Brush the inner sides of the teeth also, and take out all bits of food from between them with a wooden tooth-pick. When this is not done, these little particles decay and make the breath very offensive. In cleaning your teeth use tepid water, for cold or hot water may crack the enamel.

2. Do not keep your tippet, overcoat, or sack on while indoors. If you are thoughtless about this, you will be apt to feel chilly and to take cold when you go out. Never forget to take off your rubber boots or shoes while in the school-room or in the house at home. Rubbers make your stockings wet with perspiration, and then when you go out of doors you are apt to take cold.

3. You should change all your clothing on going to bed. The clothing worn next to your skin should be aired and dried at night, and should be well shaken before it is put on again in the morning.

4. If your clothing gets wet in a storm, don't stand or sit still and shiver, but keep moving to keep warm till you can take off the wet clothing. You should not sit in school with wet clothing or wet feet. Severe sickness may be caused by so doing.

5. Try to have regular hours for work, play, and sleep. Plenty of exercise and plenty of rest in sleep, if taken at right times, make bright minds and strong bodies. While we sleep the brain rests, and even the heart works a little slower and gets rested.

6. Children need more sleep than grown-up people. Those who sit up late at night have pale faces, dull brains, and weak bodies. The brain and the nerves must have plenty of rest in sleep, or they will soon wear out. Children who play hard and study hard should have all the sleep they can take.

7. Try to remember all that you have read in this little book, and practise what you have learned about keeping good health. God has given you these wonderful bodies to take care of; and it is your duty to try to become strong, healthy men and women, so that you can be happy and useful in the world.

TEST QUESTIONS FOR REVIEW.

EYESIGHT AND HEARING.—HEALTH HINTS.

Lesson XXVI. — Where are our eyes placed, and how are they guarded? How does light get into our eyes? Tell about the screen that regulates the light. Where does the light go at last, and what then? Tell what good eyes can do. What is said about the sight of old people? What trouble have many children in seeing? What rules have you learned for taking care of your sight? Where are the parts of your ears that do the hearing? Tell about the tube of the ear and the drum-head. What is the use of the ear-wax? Why is it dangerous to pick at your ears? If anything gets into your ear, what should you do? What about shouting into anybody's ears?

Lesson XXVII. — How do alcohol and tobacco harm the eyes? What harm does cigarette smoking do to the eyes? In what other way do alcohol and tobacco injure eyesight? What would pure alcohol do to the mouth and throat? How may strong liquors injure good hearing?

Lesson XXVIII. — How often should your teeth be cleaned? Tell how to brush the teeth best. Tell about taking bits of food from between them, and why. Why should you not wear tippets, overcoats, and sacks while in-doors? Tell about wearing rubbers while in-doors. What have you read about changing your clothing on going to bed? How should you care for your day clothing? What is said about wearing wet clothing? About wet feet in school? What is said about exercise and sleep? Why should children have plenty of sleep? Tell what is said about sitting up late. What is your duty to your bodies, and why?

www.ingramcontent.com/pod-product-compliance
Lightning Source LLC
Chambersburg PA
CBHW031440270326
41930CB00007B/805